HOMEMADE MEDICAL FACE MASK

The Ultimate Step-by-Step Guide to Make Easily and Quickly Your Diy Medical Mask at Home for Protection Against Disease, Viruses, Germs, Bacteria and Flu.

DAVID WHITE

© **Copyright 2019 –David White All rights reserved.**

The content contained within this book may not be reproduced, duplicated or transmitted without direct written permission from the author or the publisher.

Under no circumstances will any blame or legal responsibility be held against the publisher, or author, for any damages, reparation, or monetary loss due to the information contained within this book. Either directly or indirectly.

Legal Notice:

This book is copyright protected. This book is only for personal use. You cannot amend, distribute, sell, use, quote or paraphrase any part, or the content within this book, without the consent of the author or publisher.

Disclaimer Notice:

Please note the information contained within this document is for educational and entertainment purposes only. All effort has been executed to present accurate, up to date, and reliable, complete information. No warranties of any kind are declared or implied. Readers acknowledge that the author is not engaging in the rendering of legal, financial, medical or professional advice. The content within this book has been derived from various sources. Please consult a licensed professional before attempting any techniques outlined in this book.

By reading this document, the reader agrees that under no circumstances is the author responsible for any losses, direct or indirect, which are incurred as a result of the use of information contained within this document, including, but not limited to, — errors, omissions, or inaccuracies.

TABLE OF CONTENTS

Chapter 1: What Is Face Mask? 1

Chapter 2: Technical Markers Of A Decent Face Veil 7

Chapter 3: How To Appropriately Wear A Face Cover And When To Wear A Face Veil? 13

Chapter 4: Precaution For The Use Of Clinical Face Veil And Types Masks 16

Chapter 5: Type Of Face Veils 19

Chapter 6: How To Appropriately Wear A Face Veil And When To Wear A Face Cover? 22

Chapter 7: Precaution For The Utilization Of Clinical Face Cover And Types Masks 25

Chapter 8: How To Make Medical Homemade Face Mask (Include Illustrations) 28

CHAPTER 1
WHAT IS FACE MASK?

Cautious spread

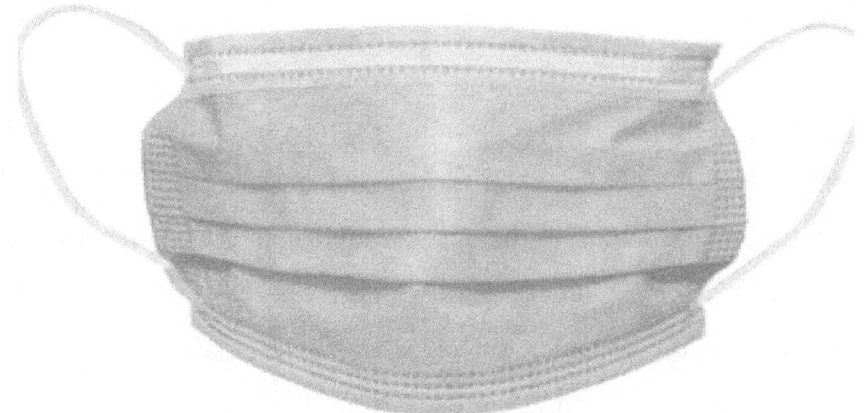

A cautious spread, in any case, called a system cloak, clinical shroud or fundamentally as a face spread, is relied upon to be worn by prosperity specialists during a clinical method and during nursing to get the infinitesimal life forms to shed in liquid globules and pressurized canned items from the wearer's mouth and nose. They are not planned to shield the wearer from taking in airborne tiny creatures or disease particles and are less convincing than respirators, for instance, N or FFP covers, which give better confirmation given their material, shape and tight seal. Cautious spreads are broadly worn by the general populace all through the whole year in East Asian countries like China, Japan,

South Korea, and Taiwan to reduce the chance of spreading airborne disorders to others, and to hinder the taking in of airborne buildup particles made using air tainting. Likewise, the cautious cloak has become a structure announcement, particularly in contemporary East Asian culture bolstered by its commonness in Japanese and Korean standard society which bigly influences East Asian youth culture.

Limit

A cautious cloak is a loose, unimportant contraption that makes a physical limit between the mouth and nose of the wearer and potential contaminants in the speedy condition. At whatever point worn properly, a cautious spread is proposed to help square tremendous atom globules, sprinkles, showers, or splatter that may contain diseases and minute creatures, protecting it from showing up at the wearer's mouth and nose. The cautious cover may in like manner help decrease the introduction of the wearer's salivation and respiratory emanations to other people. Careful spread moreover reminds wearers not to contact their mouth or nose, which could by one way or another move diseases and microorganisms in the wake of having reached a contaminated surface. A cautious cloak, by design, doesn't channel or square little particles recognizable all around that may be transmitted by hacks, wheezes, or certain clinical philosophy. Cautious shroud furthermore doesn't give complete confirmation from germs and various contaminants because of the free fit between the outside of the face spread and the face. A cautious shroud isn't to be confused with a respirator and isn't confirmed in that limit. The cautious cover is not expected to shield the wearer from taking in airborne infinitesimal creatures or disease particles and are less fruitful than respirators, which are proposed for this reason. Assortment capability of cautious spread channels can go from under % to about % for different makers' spreads when evaluated using the test parameters for NIOSH affirmation. In any case, an assessment found that on any occasion, for cautious cover with "extraordinary" channels, – % of subjects bombarded an OSHA-recognized emotional fittest, and a quantitative test showed – % spillage. The present-day cautious cover is delivered utilizing paper or other non-woven material and should be discarded after each ut

ilization.

Physical structure

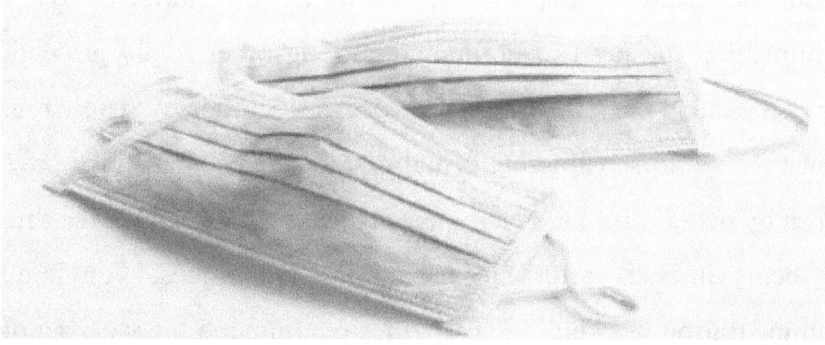

The structure of the cautious spreads depends upon the mode; ordinarily, the cloak is three-use (three layers). This three-utilize material is comprised of a break down blown material put between the non-woven surface. The mellowed blown material goes about as the channel that keeps life forms from entering or leaving the cover.

The most cautious cover incorporates wrinkles or overlays. Three wrinkles are used to allow the customer to develop the shroud with the ultimate objective that it covers the domain from the nose to the stunning. There are three exceptional ways to deal with ensuring the cover. The most notable is the ear circle, where a string-like material is attached to the spread and put behind the ears. The other is the tie-on, which involves four non-woven lashes that are tied behind the head. The third is the headband, an adaptable tie that is ensured about behind the head.

Use

A cautious spread, or technique cover, is proposed to be worn by prosperity specialists during a clinical method and certain human administration systems to get microorganisms shed in liquid globules and pressurized canned items from the wearer's mouth and nose. Verification supports the feasibility of cautious cover in diminishing the peril of defilement among other social protection workers and in the network. In any case, a Cochrane overview found that there is no sensible confirmation that unnecessary face covers worn by people from the cautious gathering would reduce the threat of bent illnesses after clean cautious techniques. For human administration workers, security rules recommend the wearing of a face-fit attempted N or FFP respirator spread instead of a cautious cover in the locale of pandemic-flu patients, to diminish the nearness of the wearer to perhaps compelling fog concentrates and airborne liquid beads.

By and large populace

In social order and home settings, the usage of facemasks and respirators overall is not recommended, with various assessments supported, for instance, dodging close contact and keeping up incredible hand cleanliness. Cautious spreads are pervasively worn by the general populace all through the whole year in East Asian countries like China, Japan, South Korea, and Taiwan to decrease the chance of spreading airborne diseases to others, and to prevent the taking in of airborne buildup particles made utilizing air contamination. In Japan and Taiwan, it isn't sudden to see these cover worn during this present season's influenza infection season, as a showing of suspected for others and social obligation. Careful spreads give some confirmation against the spread of infections, and improvised spreads give about half as much insurance. A few countries like Slovakia introduced required covers out in the open vehicle and open spaces during the coronavirus pandemic. Even more starting late, as a result of the rising issue of darker fog in South and Southeast Asia, cautious spreads and an air isolating face covers are directly a great part of the time used in critical urban territories in India, Nepal, and Thailand when air quality disintegrates to destructive levels. Moreover, face covers are used in Indonesia, Malaysia, and Singapore during the Southeast Asian obscurity season. Besides, cautious spreads have become a style clarification, particularly in contemporary East Asian culture bolstered by its unmistakable quality in Japanese and Korean standard society which bigly influences East Asian youth culture air filtering cautious style cloak is very notable across Asia and in this manner, various associations have released covers that not simply prevent the taking in of airborne buildup particles and yet are chic. Careful spreads with excellent plans are celebrated in countries in which they are worn openly. Cautious spreads may moreover be worn to mask character. In the United States banks, comfort stores, etc have confined their use as a result of criminals on and on doing accordingly. In the – Hong Kong battles, some protestors wore cautious spreads among various sorts of the cloak to avoid affirmation, and the organization endeavored to blacklist such use.

Rule

In the United States, the cautious cover is cleared for advancing by the U.S. Sustenance and Drug Administration. Beginning in, producers of cautious cloak must show that their thing is on any occasion on a standard with a spread starting at now accessible to procure "breathing space" for displaying. Makers may investigate channel tests using a characteristic living being airborne, or a disintegrated of.

CHAPTER 2
TECHNICAL MARKERS OF A DECENT FACE VEIL

Establishment

Since certain unimportant filtering facepiece particulate respirators are tantamount in appearance to various cautious/methodology cover, their aberrations are not for each situation unquestionably known. In any case, respirators and cautious/procedure cloak are through and through various in anticipated use, fit against the face, wear time, testing and underwriting. The purpose behind this chronicle is to highlight a portion of these qualifications, particularly for restorative administration workers. Cautious/framework spreads may be given to patients to help guarantee human administration workers and various patients from particles being brought into the room as a patient talks, wheezes or hacks.

Wear Time

Respirators must be fittingly picked and carefully wore (put on) and doffed (taken off) in an immaculate district, and worn the entire time in the corrupted domain to altogether influence the diminishing presentation. Having the respirator off even 10% of the time in a spoiled region lessens the guarded effect of the respirator. Cautious/technique shroud are regularly worn (put on) for a specific

7

procedure. For infection control purposes, the cloak is conventionally disposed of after each method/tolerant development.

Testing

In the United States, respirators must meet test criteria communicated in the Code of Federal Regulations 42 CFR Part 84. For a total appreciation of all the test criteria, the per-client should review the rules. The channel capability test criteria, which are used by the U.S. National Institute for Occupational Safety and Health (NIOSH), for respirators with "N95" channel media include:

• Sodium chloride test disintegrated with a mass center streamlined broadness (MMAD) atom of about 0.3 μm;

• Airflow pace of 85 liters for every minute (ppm);

• Charge-slaughtered test disintegrated; and

• Preconditioning at 85% relative dampness (RH) and 38°C for 24 hours before testing. Normal tests for cautious/procedure shroud incorporate atom filtration adequacy (PFE), bacterial filtration capability (BFE), fluid check, differential weight, and instability. Each test is immediately delineated underneath.

Particulate Filtration Efficiency (PFE)

The PFE test is a quality pointer for social protection cautious/strategy covers. The PFE test isn't a pointer of respirator affirmation execution. The channel media of a cautious/methodology spread with an incredibly high (>95%) PFE may by the by be under 70% beneficial when attempted with the

NIOSH N95 test procedure. The eventual outcomes of the cautious/approach shroud PFE testing and NIOSH filtration adequacy testing should not be broke down. Conditions of the PFE test include:

- Polystyrene latex circle test disintegrated;
- Approximately 0.1 µm in size;
- Airflow pace of 28 liters for every minute (ppm);
- Un-slaughtered test disintegrated; and
- No preconditioning

Bacterial Filtration Efficiency (BFE)

This test overviews the limit of a cautious/technique spread to give a limit to enormous particles evacuated by the wearer. It's not a substitute for a managerial respirator filtration viability test and it doesn't evaluate the cautious/technique spread's ability to give any security to the wearer. The test technique used to evaluate BFE is the American Society of Testing and Materials (ASTM) methodology F2101-01.

Fluid Resistance

The fluid obstacle test is normally coordinated reliant on the ASTM Test Method F 1862, "Assurance from Penetration by Manufactured Blood," which chooses the spread's insurance from designed blood squirted at it under fluctuating loads. Differential Pressure (Delta-P)

The Delta-P test is routinely driven reliant on the "Procedure 1 Military Specifications: Surgical Mask, nonessential (June 12, 1975)", MIL-M-36945C 4.4.1.1.1. Delta-P is the conscious weight drop over the cautious/technique spread material besides, it is related to the cover's breathability.

Imperviousness to fire

Cautious/technique covers expected to be used in the working room experience testing to choose the instability by class. FDA endorses that Class 1 and Class 2 instability materials be used. The U.S. Sustenance and Drug Administration (FDA) endorses the usage of one of the rules underneath to test instability.

- UL 2154 End

With everything taken into account, cautious/strategy shroud are proposed to help put a deterrent between the wearer and the work environment or sterile field. They may help keep with spitting and mucous made by the wearer from showing up at a patient or clinical apparatus. They can moreover be used as fluid prevention to help keep with blooding splatter from showing up at the wearer's mouth and nose. Regardless, cautious/technique cloak can't give affirmed respiratory protection aside from on the off chance that they are similarly arranged, attempted, and government-affirmed as a respirator. If a wearer needs to diminish the internal breath of humbler, inhalable particles (those more diminutive than 100 microns), they need to procure and properly use an organization affirmed respirator, for instance, a NIOSH-ensured N95 filtering facepiece particulate respirator. If the wearer needs a mix cautious/strategy spread and a particulate respirator, they ought to use a thing that is both cleared by FDA as a cautious/technique cover and attempted and guaranteed by NIOSH as a particulate respirator. Such things are on occasion called a "clinical respirator," "therapeutic administration respirator," or "cautious N95." Respirator versus Surgical/Procedure Mask Decision Tree for Healthcare Workers The going with decision tree highlights potential examinations for the assurance of respirators segments cautious/strategy shroud.

• The selection of respiratory protection for word related dangers is normally established on the airborne centralization of the substance that the wearer is introduced to and the word related introduction limit (OEL) of that substance.

• Biological administrators, for instance, diseases and minute life forms, don't have OELs; as needs are, supervisors should think about available heading while at the same time picking respirators. The U.S. Networks for Disease Control and Prevention (CDC) has recommended that respirators offering more confirmation, for instance, controlled air cleansing respirators (PAPRs), may be considered in conditions right when high exposures to microorganisms and contaminations are possible.

• The word related to the use of respirators in the U.S. is overseen by the U.S. Word related Safety and Health Administration (OSHA), and in the U.S., the use of respirators in every workplace must be per OSHA standard 29 CFR 1910.134.

• Tight-fitting respirators, for instance, extra isolating facepiece particulate respirators can't be worn with facial hair or whatever else that may intrude with the seal of the respirator to the wearer's face.

CHAPTER 3
HOW TO APPROPRIATELY WEAR A FACE COVER AND WHEN TO WEAR A FACE VEIL?

Wearing Mask

Why wear a spread?

Extraordinary Acute Respiratory Syndrome (SARS) can be transmitted by respiratory dots over a short partition or through direct contact with a patient's outflows. Wearing a cover offers protection from SARS. If you have a respiratory tract malady, it also prevents the spread of the ailment. Cautious shroud, if suitably worn, is convincing in preventing the spread of globule ailments.

Wearing a spread is just one way to deal with assistance thwart respiratory tract defilements. Most huge is to watch worthy individual tidiness. Wash hands as regularly as conceivable with the liquid chemical. Ceaselessly wash turns in the wake of wheezing, hacking, cleaning the nose; taking off to the can; and before reaching the eyes, nose, and mouth, or arranging sustenance. You can in like manner create body insusceptibility by working up a strong lifestyle - eat well, get a ton of rest, work out, don't smoke.

Who should wear a cloak?

People with respiratory illness symptoms: Individuals who care for patients with respiratory infection reactions. People who have been in close contact with insisted or suspected SARS patients should wear a spread for at any rate 10 days from the last contact.

People visiting focuses or facilities

Human administration workers in clinical settings. Workers dealing with sustenance, Open vehicle operational staff Individuals in swarmed or ineffectually ventilated spots. Understudies and staff at schools (Aside from during physical preparing practices or in an inside and out ventilated and broad setting with no "short division eye to eye development" included) As this summary can't be complete, people from individuals, by and large, are reminded to rehearse judgment following the bearing given beforehand. All things considered, any person who needs to wear a spread is urged to do thusly. Persistently keep a cover accommodating with the objective that you can put one on as the need arises. Centers to note about wearing a spread:

Wash hands before putting on a spread, when taking an interesting case. Hold fast to the bearings given by the supplier. When wearing a cautious shroud, ensure that: The cover fits comfortably over the face. The toned side of the cloak faces outwards, with the metallic strip most elevated. The strings or adaptable gatherings are arranged fittingly to keep the cloak emphatically set up. The shroud covers the nose, mouth, and stunning. The metallic strip molds to the platform of the nose. Reach the spread once it is ensured pretty much all over as ceaseless dealing with may decrease its confirmation. In case you ought to do, all things considered, wash your hands while reaching the cloak When expelling the shroud, swear off reaching the outside of the spread as this part may be made sure about with germs.

In the wake of evacuating the spread, overlay the cloak outwards (for instance the outside of the spread standing up to inwards), by then put the shroud into a plastic or paper sack before putting it into a decline container with a top. A cautious cloak should be discarded after use and in no way, shape or form should it be used for longer than a day. Override the spread rapidly on the off chance that it is hurt or dirtied.

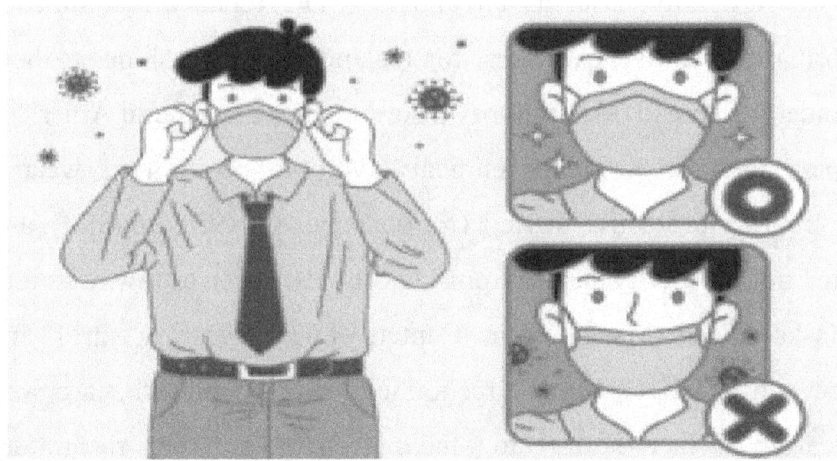

CHAPTER 4
PRECAUTION FOR THE USE OF CLINICAL FACE VEIL AND TYPES MASKS

N95 Respirators Not for Use by the Public

The Centers for Disease Control and Prevention (CDC) doesn't endorse that the general populace wears N95 respirators to shield themselves from respiratory afflictions, including coronavirus (COVID-19). The best way to deal with prevent affliction is to refrain from being introduced to this disease. In any case, as an update, CDC reliably recommends normal preventive exercises, for instance, hand washing, to help hinder the spread of respiratory disorders. For the general American open, there is no extra clinical favorable position to wear a respiratory protective device, (for instance, an N95 respirator), and the brief prosperity danger from COVID-19 is seen as low. Cautious Masks (Face Masks) The Centers for Disease Control and Prevention (CDC) doesn't recommend that people who are well wearing a face spread to shield themselves from respiratory contaminations, including coronavirus (COVID-19). A cautious spread is a loose, superfluous contraption that makes a physical limit between the mouth and nose of the wearer and potential contaminants in the brief condition. The cautious cloak is coordinated under 21 CFR 878.4040. The cautious cloak is not to be shared and may be named as cautious, disengagement, dental, or clinical framework covers. They may go with or without a face shield. These are now and again suggested as face shroud, even though not all face covers are overseen as cautious spreads. The cautious shroud is made in different thicknesses and with different abilities to shield you from contact with liquids. These properties may in like manner impact how viably you can breathe in through the face cloak and how well the cautious spread makes sure about you. At whatever point worn fittingly, a cautious cloak is planned to help square tremendous atom globules, sprinkles, showers, or splatter that may contain germs (diseases and infinitesimal creatures), protecting it from showing up at your mouth and nose. The cautious shroud may moreover help reduce the presentation of your spit and respiratory outflows to others. While a cautious spread may be incredible in blocking sprinkles and tremendous atom dots, a face cloak, by arrangement, doesn't channel or square little particles observable all around that may be transmitted by hacks, wheezes, or certain clinical system. Cautious cloak moreover doesn't give absolute confirmation from germs and various contaminants because of the free fit between the outside of the face spread and your face. The cautious cover is not wanted to be used more than once. In case your spread is hurt or dirtied, or if breathing through the cloak gets problematic, you ought to oust the face shroud, discard it safely, and displace it with another. To safely discard your spread, place it in a plastic sack and put it in the garbage. Wash your hands in the wake of managing the used shroud.

N95 Respirators

An N95 respirator is a respiratory cautious contraption planned to achieve an extraordinarily close facial fit and capable filtration of airborne particles. The 'N95' task suggests that when presented to mindful testing, the respirator hinders at any rate 95 percent of astoundingly little (0.3 microns) test particles. On the off chance that suitably fitted, the filtration capacities of N95 respirators outperform those of face cloak. In any case, even a suitably fitted N95 respirator doesn't discard the peril of affliction or death.

CHAPTER 5
TYPE OF FACE VEILS

1. Face Masks For Personal Use

On the off chance that you have to maintain a strategic distance from the potential danger of wearing a face spread when you're not incapacitated, the best thing you can do is make a shroud for yourself — don't get one and add to the need. We've collected some basic instructional activities here with the expectation of complimentary cloak that protected against respiratory globules. Recall that the edges of the spread should fit snuggly against the skin.

2. Face Masks For Medical Use

On the off chance that you're fit for sewing and need to help you're close by clinical facilities, you can make colossal groups of face covers at home. There are express necessities you should meet with the ultimate objective for them to be sufficient for clinical use, so guarantee you tail them. Something different, your work may be futile.

While locally built spreads can't be clinical level, the CDC finds especially made shroud like the ones underneath to be useful. It's for each situation best to contact your crisis center early to check whether they're taking blessings — a couple of territories aren't on any occasion, allowing endowments of individual cautious equipment, and others have point by point specifics for the face covers they can get. Resources, for instance, Masks For Heroes can keep you instructed about how to give.

3. Cautious cover

The cautious shroud is disposable, loose face covers that spread your nose, mouth, and facial structure. They're normally used to: shield the wearer from showers, sprinkles, and enormous atom dots thwart the spread of possibly compelling respiratory releases from the wearer to others Careful cloak can vary in structure, in any case, the spread itself is oftentimes level and rectangular alive and well with wrinkles or cover. The most elevated purpose of the cloak contains a metal strip that can be encircled to your nose. Adaptable gatherings or long, straight ties help hold a cautious spread set up while you're wearing it. These can either be hovered behind your ears or tied behind your head.

4. N95 respirators

An N95 respirator is an even more tight-fitting face cloak. Despite sprinkles, sprinkles, and enormous dots, this respirator can in like manner filter through 95 percent confided in Source of incredibly little particles. This joins diseases and microorganisms. The respirator itself is generally round or oval perfectly healthy and is expected to shape a tight seal to your face. Adaptable gatherings help hold it steadfastly to your face. A couple of sorts may have an association called an exhalation valve, which can help with breathing and the advancement of warmth and moisture. N95 respirators aren't one-size-fits-all. They should be fit-attempted before use to guarantee that a genuine seal is molded. In case the spread doesn't seal effectively to your face, you won't get the fitting security. In the wake of being fit-attempted, customers of N95 respirators must continue playing out a seal check each time they put one on. It's similarly basic to observe that a tight seal can't be cultivated in specific get-togethers. These fuse children and people with facial hair.

CHAPTER 6
HOW TO APPROPRIATELY WEAR A FACE VEIL AND WHEN TO WEAR A FACE COVER?

Wearing Mask

Why wear a spread?

Extraordinary Acute Respiratory Syndrome (SARS) can be transmitted by respiratory globules over a short partition or through direct contact with a patient's emanations. Wearing a cover offers protection from SARS. In the event that you have a respiratory tract infection, it also prevents the spread of the disorder. Cautious shroud, if fittingly worn, is convincing in preventing the spread of globule infections.

Wearing a spread is just one way to deal with assistance hinders respiratory tract pollutions. Most critical is to watch adequate individual tidiness. Wash hands as frequently as conceivable with the liquid chemical. Ceaselessly wash turns in the wake of sneezing, hacking, cleaning the nose; taking off to the can; and before reaching the eyes, nose, and mouth, or arranging sustenance. You can moreover create body immunity by working up a strong lifestyle - eat well, get a great deal of rest, work out, don't smoke.

Who should wear a cover?

People with respiratory infection reactions: Individuals who care for patients with respiratory malady symptoms. People who have been in close contact with certified or suspected SARS patients should wear a spread for at any rate 10 days from the last contact.

People visiting focuses or centers

Human administration workers in clinical settings. Workers dealing with sustenance, Open vehicle operational staff Individuals in swarmed or incapably ventilated spots. Understudies and staff at schools (Aside from during physical preparing practices or in an inside and out ventilated and broad setting with no "short division eye to eye development" included) As this overview can't be thorough, people from individuals, when all is said in done, are reminded to rehearse judgment following the heading given beforehand. All things considered, any person who needs to wear a spread is urged to do in that capacity. Consistently keep a cloak accommodating with the objective that you can put one on as the need arises. Centers to note about wearing a spread:

Wash hands before putting on a spread, when taking a one of a kind case. Cling to the bearings given by the supplier. When wearing a cautious cover, ensure that: The shroud fits comfortably over the face. The tinted side of the cloak faces outwards, with the metallic strip most noteworthy. The strings or adaptable gatherings are arranged fittingly to keep the cover positively set up. The cloak covers the nose, mouth, and stunning. The metallic strip molds to the platform of the nose. Reach the spread once it is ensured pretty much all over as ceaseless dealing with may decrease its confirmation. If you ought to do, all things considered, wash your hands while reaching the shroud When evacuating the cloak, keep away from reaching the outside of the spread as this part may be made sure about with germs.

In the wake of expelling the spread, overlay the cloak outwards (for instance the outside of the spread standing up to inwards), by then put the shroud into a plastic or paper sack before setting it into a deny container with a top. A cautious cover should be discarded after use and in no way, shape or form should it be used for longer than a day. Supersede the spread rapidly on the off chance that it is hurt or dirtied.

CHAPTER 7
PRECAUTION FOR THE UTILIZATION OF CLINICAL FACE COVER AND TYPES MASKS

N95 Respirators Not for Use by the Public

The Centers for Disease Control and Prevention (CDC) doesn't endorse that the general populace wears N95 respirators to shield themselves from respiratory disorders, including coronavirus (COVID-19). The best way to deal with hinder sickness is to swear off being introduced to this disease. In any case, as an update, CDC reliably endorses standard preventive exercises, for instance, hand washing, to help hinder the spread of respiratory disorders. For the general American open, there is no extra clinical bit of leeway to wear a respiratory cautious device, (for instance, an N95 respirator), and the brief prosperity peril from COVID-19 is seen as low. Cautious Masks (Face Masks) The Centers for Disease Control and Prevention (CDC) doesn't recommend that people who are well wearing a face spread to shield themselves from respiratory contaminations, including coronavirus (COVID-19). A cautious spread is a loose, nonessential contraption that makes a physical limit between the mouth and nose of the wearer and potential contaminants in the brief condition. Cautious cover are coordinated under 21 CFR 878.4040. The cautious cloak is not to be shared and may be named as cautious, withdrawal, dental, or clinical framework covers. They may go with or without a face shield. These are habitually suggested as face shroud, in spite of the fact that not all face covers are overseen as cautious spreads. The cautious cloak is made in different thicknesses and with different abilities to shield you from contact with liquids. These properties may in like manner impact how viably you can breathe in through the face cloak and how well the cautious spread makes sure about you. At whatever point worn fittingly, a cautious shroud is expected to help square enormous particle dots, sprinkles, showers, or splatter that may contain germs (contaminations and minuscule living beings), protecting it from showing up at your mouth and nose. Cautious cloak may similarly help decrease the presence of your spit and respiratory emanations to others. While a cautious spread may be incredible in blocking sprinkles and tremendous atom dabs, a face cover, by setup, doesn't channel or square little particles recognizable all around that may be transmitted by hacks, wheezes, or certain clinical technique. Cautious cloak moreover doesn't give absolute affirmation from germs and various contaminants because of the free fit between the outside of the face spread and your face. The cautious cover is not intended to be used more than once. In case your spread is hurt or dirtied, or if breathing through the shroud gets inconvenient, you ought to remove the face cloak, discard it safely, and override it with another. To safely discard your spread, place it in a plastic sack and put it in the garbage. Wash your hands in the wake of managing the used cover.

N95 Respirators

An N95 respirator is a respiratory guarded contraption proposed to achieve an extraordinarily close facial fit and capable filtration of airborne particles. The 'N95' task infers that when presented to wary testing, the respirator deters at any rate 95 percent of incredibly little (0.3 microns) test particles. In the event that suitably fitted, the filtration capacities of N95 respirators outperform those of face shroud. In any case, even a properly fitted N95 respirator doesn't discard the threat of affliction or end.

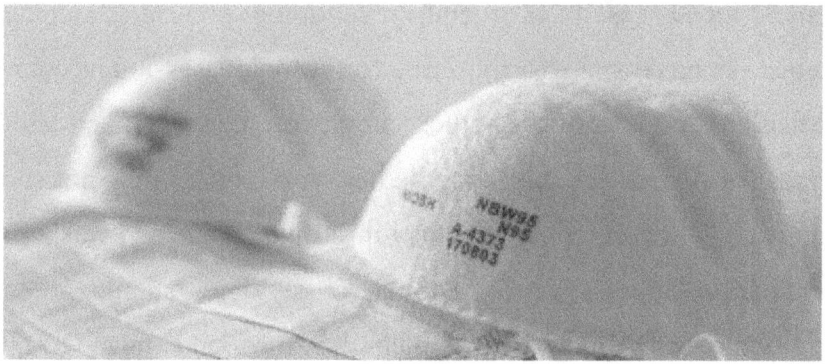

CHAPTER 8
HOW TO MAKE MEDICAL HOMEMADE FACE MASK (INCLUDE ILLUSTRATIONS)

Bit by bit directions to Sew a Face Mask

Bearing on whether to wear a face cover has been creating. The Centers for Disease Control and Prevention at present admonishes against strong people wearing shroud anyway is assessing its course, particularly considering another conviction that as much as 25 percent of people debased with the new coronavirus may not show signs. It is still commonly basic to limit trips outside and wash your hands from time to time. Customary individuals should not use clinical assessment covers, which are rare and must be put something aside for therapeutic administration workers on the front line. Regardless, the people who are cleared out with the new coronavirus can help limit the spread of respiratory globules by wearing a cover, and that applies to the people who are asymptomatic or unfamiliar as well. Moreover, a couple of affiliations are using the surface shroud as a fleeting stopgap.

You will require:

Devices

Needle and string (and a sewing machine, on the off chance that you have one)

Scissors

Pins or fastens to hold surfaces set up (self catching pins and paper catches will in like manner work after every single other choice have been depleted)

Materials

In any occasion 20 by 20 drags of 100 percent cotton surface, for instance, a level tea towel

4 bits of cotton surface forties, around 18" long and ¾" wide

Or then again

4 level, clean shoelaces

Set up YOUR MATERIALS

Stage 1

Pick your bit of cotton surface, prewash it on the most sweltering setting and dry it on high warmth. (Tea towels are more intelligent to use than T-shirts or materials, according to the Stanford Anesthesia Informatics and Media Lab.) Overlay the surface down the center. Measure and cut out a 9.5" by 6.5" square shape to make two vaguely evaluated layers. This is your shroud base.

Cut 4 slim bits of material, around 18" long and ¾" wide, Cover each piece of surface twice longwise, by then again to overlap the unforgiving edges inside. Sew a straight line along the middle. This will thwart the surface ties from having frayed edges.

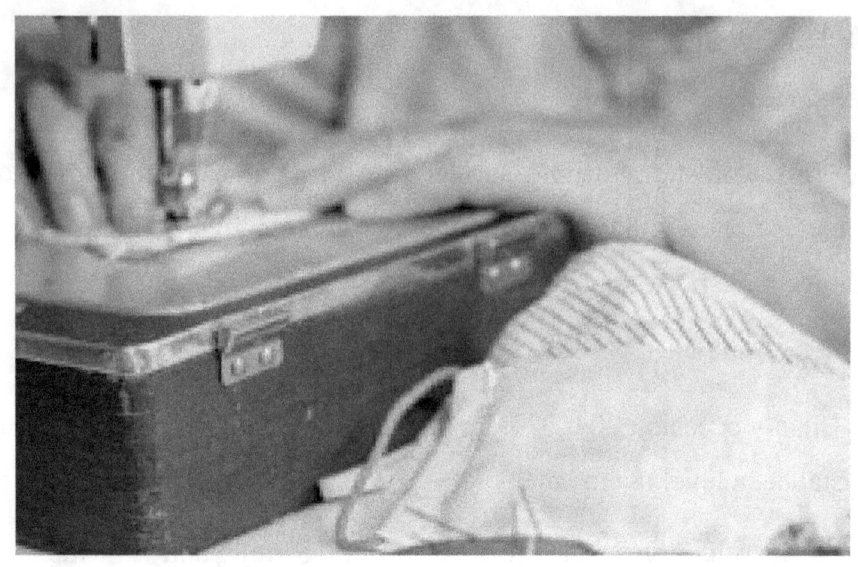

Counting THE TIES

Stage 2

Take one of your rectangular surface layers. With the "right side" (or the outer standing up to the side, where the model perhaps) facing you, nail down the 4 surface ties, one piece for each corner. Guarantee that the ties are collected in the point of convergence of the surface layer before advancing to the accompanying stage. You can similarly substitute sewing adaptable for surface ties, yet note that flexible can't be blurred (and right now, easy to clean) and that anyone with a latex excessive touchiness can't wear it. (Adaptable is in like manner dynamically difficult to find.) Attach elastics to the chief layer of a surface by ensuring about the terminations at the corners, surrounding little groups. Guarantee the adaptable lies inside the edge of your surface.

Amassing IT

Stage 3

Take the second layer of the surface and line it up with the first. The "right sides" (or planned sides) of the surface should face each other, sandwiching the surface ties or elastics. Secure the surface sandwich together with pins.

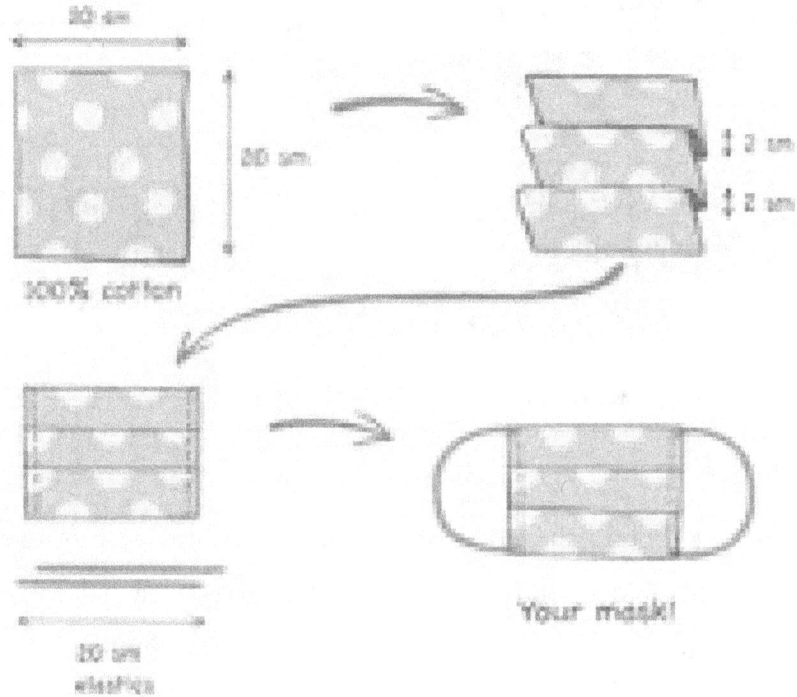

Start STITCHING

Stage 4

Eyeball a midpoint. From the middle, sew a straight line over the cover, about ¼" over the base edge of the surface, near the base left-hand corner. Oust any pins as you sew past them. Guarantee that the adaptable or surface ties are ensured about in the corners, sandwiched by your two layers of surface, as you sew over their completions. You have to guarantee your needle encounters the three pieces: the top layer, the completion of the surface tie, and the base layer. Incorporate a few join forward and in switch (in the two headings) to ensure about your ties set up.

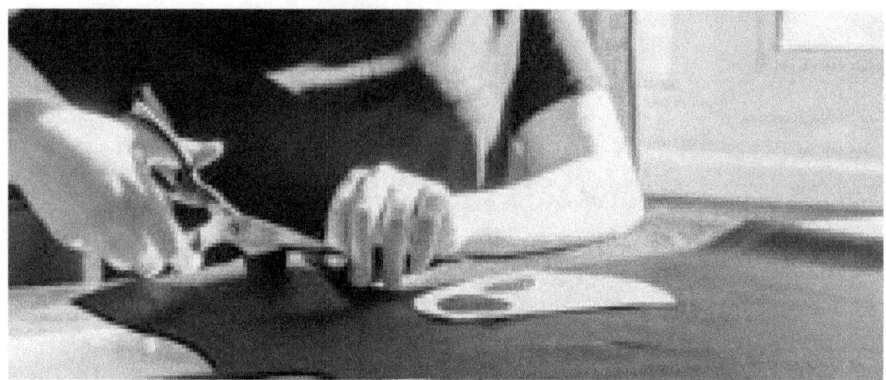

Line ALL AROUND

Stage 5

Line all around the edge of the surface layers, repeating the development and in the opposite development at each corner to ensure pretty much all the flexible completions or surface ties continue sewing your way at the starting stage, yet stop to contemplate a 1 ½" hole.

TURN OUT

Stage 6

Turn your assignment right-side-out from the little 1 ½" gap. Your surface ties or elastics should now stick out, like little legs.

Stage 7

Make three dazed wrinkles the long route on the cloak, just as crumbling a paper fan. This makes the cover change in accordance with the wearer's face. Secure each wrinkle with pins.

Wrapping UP

Stage 8

With your wrinkles held set up by pins, join around the fringe of the spread, ¼" away from the edge of the wrinkle. This is known as the top line. Take care when sewing over the wrinkles as the surface may be exceptionally thick. To affix a second time around, about ¼" in from the first round of sewing by and by you have a completed cloak, Next up? Making sense of how to wear a cloak viably is noteworthy. Various people pull them aside, hampering their effect, and, air can get in actuality around the edges.

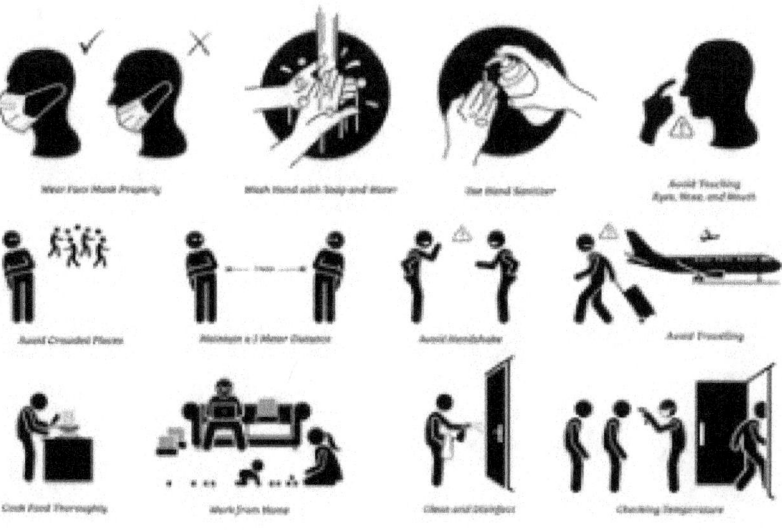

www.ingramcontent.com/pod-product-compliance
Lightning Source LLC
Chambersburg PA
CBHW050307220526
45465CB00002B/857